Also by Wanda Bailey

Divorce Blueprint

Going Gluten Free

www.mydivorceblueprint.com

www.mommywisesup.com

www.dragongempublishing.com

WEIGHT LOSS BACK 2 BASICS

By Wanda Bailey

The Stripped Down Naked Truth About Dieting and Why Your Diet Doesn't Work

WEIGHT LOSS BACK 2 BASICS
Second Edition
Published by Dragon Gem Publishing
Copyright © 2015 by Wanda Bailey
Cover by Wanda Bailey

Contents

Preface

If you've bought this book – or are thinking about buying this book – you're struggling. You've been struggling. This may be the first time you've struggled with your weight (if so – you're lucky). This may be the umpteenth time you've struggled with your weight.

You may have come to the slow realization that the weight loss industry – is not your friend. Oh, they're friendly, all right. They are more than happy to flood your television, your e-mail and your mailbox with helpful tips and tricks on how to lose weight and keep it off. And you keep getting those e-mails, and magazines, and watching those television shows, and buying those videos, and visiting those shelves at Wal-mart and CVS watching for the next great gadget or pill or drink that's going to solve your problem.

I know – I've been there. I've done that. I've stretched the t-shirt, I've bagged it. I've spent the equivalent of a small island's gross domestic annual production on finding the solution.

But you know what – I've known the solution all along. And so have you. It's to… wait for it… we have to eat less. Surprised? Shocked? You shouldn't be. You've known it all along, haven't you? In this day and age of Super-Size Me, our portions and proportions have grown epically. Medical researchers are getting in on the business now, and spending millions of research dollars on the "obesity epidemic" – dollars that could be spent to cure cancer and other diseases.

We, as a nation, eat too much. Our restaurants serve too much. We snack too much. Fifty years ago, we had smaller plates, smaller cups, we were smaller people. Now look at us.

So what do we do? We have to eat less. But…but – we want more! Yeah, I know. Sigh. I want more, too. But I want to have a normal sized body, a body that will last long enough to see a grandchild, a great-grandchild. And to do that – I have to down-size. So walk with me through this – instead of the Super-size Me, let's, all of us – Minimize Me, and get Back 2 Basics!

*Special Note – What is the Venus Factor Program?

Scattered throughout this book, I'll be talking about the Venus Factor program, and referring to the Venus members. <u>Yes – it's a paid "weight loss industry" deal</u>. But here's why I like it – it has a one-time price, but you get to access the member forums and updates for LIFE. (Or as long as the business model keeps it going, and as far as I can see, it's going pretty well!) For a one-time fee of $47.00 USD, you get the food/eating program, the exercise program with videos, and the member forums and blogs. (You will be offered up-sells – I'd turn them down. Also – un-subscribe from their e-mails as quickly as possible, they'll flood you with additional "buy-me" products – more "diet industry" money wasters and gimmicks and "never eat these 5 foods" junk advice). The Forums are a hoot – women just like you and me, they're successful, they fail, they fall off of the wagon, they get back on it. They have lives, they're married, they're single, they're healthy, they're sick, they have auto-immune diseases, they're at home moms, they travel for work – they're all of us. Go meet them…

Not sure about Venus Factor? You can go listen to some of the Venus Index podcasts on iTunes for free. These are interviews with some of the periodic winners (these are members that went through the program and reached their goals and submitted picture proof and were judged against other members that did the same) about how they used the program to fit with their own lifestyle needs. The Venus program is VERY flexible – there are suggested food plans, but you can really do whatever you want within the guidelines.

If you are interested in viewing more, please visit www.mommywisesup.com – Products for more information.

The Venus Factor program was conceived and marketed by John Barban. John's formal education background is a degree in human biology and nutrition from the University of Guelph (Ontario Canada), and a Masters in Human Biology and Nutrition - also from the University of Guelph. He did further graduate research and taught exercise physiology at the University of Florida. He also has personal training certifications with NSCA, CSCS, ACE PT, CSEP, and was at one point a certified kinesiologist. That being said – the guys knows exercise and nutrition.

The program he and his colleagues designed have swept the nation and revolutionized the weight loss industry. People have become fed up with the endless buzz of fad weight loss – it's refreshing to get back to the basics brought to us by Jack LaLanne in the 1950's – healthy eating and healthy exercise. Watching what we eat, and strengthening our bodies is the key to physical beauty and long, healthy lives.

ONE

How Much Should You Eat?

How much should you eat? That's a really great question! And if I was one of the popular diet gurus, I'd be advising you to eat everything you want of THIS food, but avoid THESE FIVE FOODS to LOSE WEIGHT! (Yes, I got that e-mail, too!) But the real answer is simple biology and mathematics.

Your body needs a measured amount of energy to function (calories), and it needs <u>more</u> if you exercise, or are pregnant or nursing. You can find a lot of websites on the internet to measure that instantly – but if you use the MyFitnessPal app, it will do it on your smart phone. It takes into account your height, current weight, age, and gender, and voila – it gives you a calorie count. For instance, a woman that is 5' 4" tall, 40 years old that weighs 160 pounds – needs 1381 calories a day to MAINTAIN her weight. Yes, that's right – MAINTAIN. If she sits at home and does nothing, 1381 calories a day. (Pretty disheartening, right?)

But – if that woman walks around, does errands, has kids, does a workout, maybe does some yoga or strength training – her calorie requirements go up by around 500 calories. Still with me? So now, she can eat around 1800 calories to MAINTAIN her body weight. EVERY DAY she can 1800 calories.

But wait – a lot of diets are recommending that we eat… 1400 to 1800 calories a day to lose weight – ummmm… is this a joke? No, this is not a joke. The diet industry is tricking you. Day after day, year after year. They're inflating the calorie counts and food plans on the weight loss "diets" that they offer you – and they are keeping you fat. Yes, the food plans are delicious and nutritious – but you're not succeeding on those "diets" – because they are built to help you MAINTAIN your body weight.

Are you really shocked now? You should be. Are you scared that you're going to be starving yourself for the rest of your life? I hope not. But – you should be aware that if you REALLY WANT to lose weight, AND KEEP IT OFF – you are going to have to CHANGE YOUR LIFESTYLE, and decide that you're going to eat differently – forever. Not just a diet for now, but forever.

Example – you know all of the fitness industry divas and celebrities with slammin' figures? We all think nasty thought about them – yeah, I'd look like that if I had the money for a personal trainer and a special chef. Well – you're wrong. Those folks – they've figured out the secret already. THEY EAT LESS THAN EVERYONE ELSE MOST OF THE TIME. Not all of the time – just most of the time. It's not a special cook, or a special workout. It's because they just eat less than other people.

Do you have to follow a low a calorie budget EVERY SINGLE DAY? Not really. But most days, yes. The Venus Index program gives you some great weekly guidelines that help keep your body "guessing", and keep you from getting used to the same thing day in and day out. But even common weight loss theory recommends one day a week – eat more to keep from going crazy. The one thing I will say – is don't consider that a "cheating" day. Because "cheating", by definition, is WRONG. Consider that day a relaxation day – AND CONTINUE TO COUNT ALL OF YOUR CALORIES. Instead of going crazy, eat what you would NORMALLY eat if you weren't trying to lose weight. Which means – an extra 500 to 800 calories above your normal calorie budget. If you normally practice fasting for breakfast – eat breakfast. If you normally abstain from alcohol or just have a small glass of wine, have two. If you normally have one starch serving at lunch at dinner, have an extra at each meal. Have a candy bar. Do all of this stuff, or parts of all of this stuff. Be nice to yourself. Oh – and during your regular week – if you are having 400 calorie lunches and dinners – why not have half a cup of real, full fat ice cream EVERY night? OR a glass of wine? Just asking – it wouldn't put you over 1000 calories a day, even if you had a snack during the day.

Will it be hard? Yes. Will it be worth it? Yes. Will you get to eat good stuff while you're doing these changes? Yes. If you plan for it – yes. Am I going to offer you a daily food plan? No. You know what you like to eat. You can find a calorie counter. Go measure the stuff you like, and eat less of it. Right now. And keep reading.

TWO

Weigh Yourself Regularly

Use the same scale and weigh yourself regularly.

How often is regularly? That depends! For some of us, once a week is fine. For others, our weight is a constant battle – one week can mean gaining five to seven pounds, if we're not very diligent and weigh on a daily basis!

When you weigh yourself, record it! Write it down, or record it on a smart phone app, or on a spreadsheet on your computer. If your weight varies or fluctuates over the year, it's important to keep tabs on it. You'll want to journal your weight loss progress so you'll have an accurate record of it that you can reflect back on. This will also remind you just how far you've come.

Your doctor may want to see your weight history when you go for your annual checkup, especially if you're experiencing any health issues.

When trying to lose weight you have to know when you're making progress so that you can celebrate. You also have to know when you aren't so you can make adjustments. The only way to know this is to weigh yourself on a regular basis.

You should weigh yourself at least once per week to give your body time to lose weight. Since a reasonable amount of weight loss is only two to three pounds per week you want to give yourself plenty of time to lose. Weighing too soon might not give you long enough to drop weight which could discourage you.

Also, remember to weigh yourself at the same time every time - early in the morning. This is the most accurate time of the day for weighing. And make sure to wear roughly the same type of clothing each time you weigh yourself. Clothing can easily add an additional pound or two.

If you are practicing controlled fasting, it's okay to weigh later in the morning – just whatever is convenient for you.

*Special Note – Your weight may vary due to water retention and lack of complete bowel movement by a few pounds a day. Seriously? Yes – think about it. One pound is sixteen ounces – that's two measuring cups of water. That's not a whole lot. If you eat some dense foods, it can be even less food that's weighing you down. Don't be discouraged if you "weigh" more for a couple of days after eating more calories (and you can read that as MORE FOOD). It's okay, your body will eliminate that extra stuff, and you'll be back to NORMAL – or losing.

THREE

Taking Your Body Measurements

It's also important to regularly take your body measurements whether losing weight, or maintaining weight loss. Why? So that you KNOW that you are making progress! Sometimes your scale is stubborn, and gets stuck somewhere. Your body measurements may show you progress when the scale does not.

Suggested parts to measure:

- Shoulder circumference
- Bust (Women)
- Chest (Men)
- Waist (Women & Men)
- Hips (Women)
- Upper Arm
- Thigh
- Calf

You may choose to measure all body parts weekly, or just Shoulders, Chest/Bust and Waist, then the remainder of the parts monthly - it's–up to you.

How to measure – if you use a regular seamstress tape measure, have someone help you. The act of holding the tape measure will cause some muscles to distort the measurement. Use a MyoTape if you are self-measuring. These are available from retailers and on Amazon and Ebay.

FOUR

Take Before and After Pictures to Track Your Journey

When we are trying to lose weight, we have to remain motivated. But it's very difficult to do so when we don't think we're seeing results or if we think they aren't coming fast enough. In order to keep yourself moving forward to your goal, take "before" pictures of yourself to reflect back on.

We don't' see our weight loss as easily as others do because we are constantly seeing ourselves in the mirror so there is no frame of reference. "Before" pictures give you that reference.

When you take your pictures make sure to post them somewhere that you can easily reflect on them. Not only will seeing your progress inspire you to keep going, but it will also show you how far you have already come. Trying to do so by memory just isn't effective and accurate enough. I used to carry mine in one of those plastic protective wallets that Walgreen's gives you when you get photos developed (yes, get photos developed, how archaic!)

As you lose weight, don't replace your original pictures. You need to be able to see the full effect of where you started. "Before" pictures also do something else: they give you motivation not to want to go back to the way you were before.

FIVE

Be Mindful of Your Portion Sizes

Portion control is one of the easiest ways to sabotage your eating. Even if you choose many of the right foods you can still defeat the purpose of those choices by loading up on more food than you should have.

Portion size trips a lot of people up simply because they have no idea just how much food they should be consuming. They let their eyes dictate how much they eat and before you know it they've overeaten.

When starting your weight loss journey you should probably weigh your food out so you get an accurate idea of what you should have. This especially goes for protein for which a portion equals the size of a fist. At the time of publication of this book – Amazon had a great scale on sale:

There are a couple of similar scales at your local Wal-Mart in the kitchen wares section for less than $20.00.

You'll also need a good set of measuring cups, or at least a single cup with multiple measures for partial cups. AND, measuring spoons.

Talk to a certified dietitian or your doctor to determine just how much of each food group you should be consuming in order to safely lose weight. (Please keep in mind – they may be following published guidelines that recommend eating AT or ABOVE your normal calorie needs. They may be a PART OF THE DIET INDUSTRY LIE – be nice to them, and eat healthy – but eat less if you really want to lose weight). If you're already a Venus member – consult the applicable food plan for your current Index for calorie, Protein, Carbohydrate and Fat intake guidelines.

SIX

How Walking Can Improve Your Weight Loss

Walking is one of the best ways to lose weight because it requires no equipment, it can be done anywhere, day or night, indoors or outdoors and virtually anyone can do it. One of the recent Venus Index winners lives in Germany, and typically walks five to seven miles each day!

Walking is also easy on the joints, making it tolerable for most people. Even those with certain health concerns can walk.

Because of its ease, and the fact that it is a low-impact form of exercise it makes it easy to maintain long-term.

Weight loss from walking depends on your starting weight. An average person can burn up to an additional 500 calories per day just from walking. That computes to at least a pound a week - maybe more.

Walking promotes lean muscle tissue, an essential for losing weight. The more lean muscle you accumulate, the higher your metabolism will run and the more fat your body will burn.

SEVEN

Using a Pedometer or Fitness Band to Keep Track of Your Walking Miles

Pedometers and Fitness Bands are great for counting your steps to ensure that you are getting a sufficient amount of walking in each day. They also take the guesswork out of walking by providing solid proof of your efforts.

These devices are meant to motivate people to move. Most people have no idea how very little they move in a day. A pedometer or fitness bank tracking system shows valid proof that more effort needs to be made.

What is an ideal amount of steps you should be taking to help you lose weight? Around 10,000 per day - minimum. That amount of activity will burn roughly 350 calories. Some pedometer models even count calories burned, too.

Of course, the more you walk, the better. Someone who is inactive will probably only get up to less than 5,000 steps per day.

To effectively use a pedometer, you need to set realistic goals so that you don't become overwhelmed and discouraged. Then, you have to adjust the pedometer to your specific pace so as to ensure that its measurements will be accurate.

On the other hand, a fitness band may be a bit more accurate, since it typically syncs up with your smart phone and utilizes GPS technology and gets a more accurate read on steps taken.

For those of us that are fashion mavens, a fitness band isn't very appealing. You can go on eBay and find some great additions to your band by searching for "Fitbit bling". These little pieces slide right over your fitness band and make it into attractive jewelry.

One down side to the fitness trackers for Venus members – if you are using a calorie tracker like MyFitnessPal, your fitness band app may reduce calories burned from your daily calorie count! To get around this limitation – in the Settings of the app, click Premium, and sign up. There is a monthly or annual Premium price, it may be worth it to go ahead and sign up for that to avoid the temptation of overeating on your daily calorie count. Then you can set it NOT to add extra food calories when you exercise.

EIGHT

Keep a Log or Journal of Food

In order to keep yourself motivated when you're trying to lose weight you have to be able to clearly see your progress. But just looking at yourself in the mirror every day won't work since you won't recognize changes very easily. The way around this is to document your progress.

By keeping a log or a journal of your efforts and the results, you can keep a much closer eye on how your body is changing over time. This is also an excellent way to keep yourself motivated to continue.

Journaling is easy and can be done in a handwritten form or on the computer. There are numerous web-based programs available that track your progress schedule your workouts and track your food intake. The previous chapter mentioned MyFitnessPal – it's a great way to keep track of your food eaten and calories, as well as your daily and weekly weight.

Journaling also allows you to reflect back when you hit a plateau to see where changes need to be made. You just have to be diligent about keeping the information current or it will defeat the purpose.

I've heard some people say – there's no way that I can keep track of all of my food every day, <u>give me something simpler</u>! Well – you're already doing the simpler thing, you're doing nothing, and you're overweight, because you ate too much. Simple secret, friends – <u>we have to eat less, to weigh less</u>. There's no magic pills, no magic food or magic machine that's going to change that simple fact of life. The weight loss industry takes billions of your dollars every year by making you believe that something outside of your control is the reason that you are overweight. But in most cases – there are some hormone based disease exceptions – <u>eating too much makes us fat</u>. - To avoid eating too much, you need to record what you eat. It's kind of like balancing your checkbook – you record how much money you spend, right? End of chapter.

NINE

Is Skipping Meals Okay?

You're going to hear many different opinions on this subject. Almost every fitness magazine you pick up and every single fitness diva is spouting the same thing – eat a good breakfast! Eat every three hours! Eat up to six times a day!

The problem with this – is that simply by EATING – we turn on our body's desire for more FOOD. There's been a lot of research on doing something different lately – INTERMITTENT FASTING. Oh, don't go getting upset thinking I'm about to tell you to starve yourself! Just check out THIS information:

Intermittent Fasting INCREASES:

- Insulin and Leptin sensitivity, reducing the risk of chronic disease, from diabetes to heart disease and even cancer
- Ghrelin levels, also known as "the hunger hormone", go up – and yes, you DO feel hungry. BUT – this is temporary, and is associated with increased levels of growth hormone and internally produced dopamine (makes you feel good)
- Ability to become "Fat Adapted", which increases your energy by burning stored fat.

Intermittent Fasting DECREASES:

- Triglyceride levels, decreasing your risk of heart disease.

- Inflammation and free radical damage.

- Weight gain and metabolic disease risk.

So, to try out this fasting concept, consider skipping breakfast, then eat lunch and dinner. Try to keep your eating within an 8-hour time frame every day. In the 6-8 hours that you DO eat, you want to have healthy protein, minimize your carbs like pasta and bread and potatoes and exchange them for HEALTHY fats like butter, eggs, avocado, coconut oil, olive oil and nuts. You may have noticed in recent years these are the fats that some folks are calling "flat belly fats".

This will help shift you to fat burning mode from carb burning mode. Remember it may take a few weeks, and you have to do it gradually, but once you succeed in the switch to fat burning mode, you will be easily able to fast for 14 - 18 hours, and not feel hungry. Your cravings for sugar usually disappear, and it will be much easier to stay on your food plan and achieve your ideal weight.

Keep in mind that having some morning coffee with cream – doesn't necessarily mean breaking your fast! As long as you stay under 50 calories, you'll be fine, and the fat-burning will continue for you. As you get closer to the end of your fast (around lunch time), if you begin to get a headache and feel hungry – go ahead and have some string cheese, or some other protein-based snack with a high fat content. This will help you last at least another hour or so until you eat a good, satisfying meal.

Also – utilizing a fasting program like this can allow you to maximize a lower calorie diet, and not feel starved! Think about it – skipping that 350 calorie breakfast allows you to have two BIGGER meals for lunch and dinner. You can go to bed with a full stomach – yep, I just said it! It's really okay to go to bed with a full tummy. If you don't like that feeling – then stop eating a couple of hours before bed.

The other "magical" benefit that occurs when you practice fasting, is that you will radically improve the beneficial bacteria in your gut. Why is this a good thing? Because supporting healthy gut bacteria, which actually outnumber your cells 10 to one—is one of the most important things you can do to improve your immune system so you won't get sick, or get coughs, colds and flus. You will sleep better, have more energy, have increased mental clarity and concentrate better. Essentially every aspect of your health will improve.

Does practicing intermittent fasting mean that you'll never eat breakfast again? No – the word "intermittent" means "occurring at irregular intervals". At least once a week – on the day that you choose to eat ABOVE your "losing weight" calorie budget – eat some breakfast! Eggs, bacon, toast, whatever you fancy – have that. Seriously! But record it in your food journal as calories eaten.

P.S. – You know all of those "studies" that claim that it's better to eat five or six small meals a day? Turns out – all of them weren't conducted using normal scientific protocol. More diet industry lies.

TEN

Don't Confuse Hunger With Thirst

Sometimes when we think we're hungry – we're really thirsty! How can we figure out which?

1) When was the last time you ate? Compare that time to the last time you had a drink. If it's been awhile since you've had anything to drink, have a full 8 ounce glass and give yourself at least 15 minutes to see if the water helps satiate you.

2) Eating and eating…and still feeling like you have an empty stomach? Chances are you're thirsty. Grab that glass.

3) Finally, if you have a headache and are feeling fatigued, these are warning signs that you are nearing dehydration. Make it a priority to drink more water. Of course – if you haven't eaten anything all day and it's 3:00 in the afternoon – eat something!

ELEVEN

Drinking enough water

Water is essential for life, yet most of us do not consume enough of it in a day. As a result, our bodies suffer. Being sufficiently hydrated is not only important for losing weight, it is vital.

Most people don't realize that by the time you feel thirsty, your body is already in mild dehydration. The goals is to prevent thirst, not treat it.

Experts recommended that an individual drink half of their body weight in ounces of water daily. If you exercise, you should drink more to compensate for perspiration. I recommend drinking what you feel comfortable drinking! If you feel like you have to go to the bathroom a lot – is that once an hour? I call that at excuse to get up and take a walk!

Drinking water is one of the most helpful things you can do to lose weight. It aids in digestion, helps hydrate muscles to rebuild them, ensures healthy tissue, and improves circulation. Sufficient water helps organs perform properly and many other functions. But when losing weight, water is essential for helping the kidneys and digestive system to flush toxins out of the body as fat is broken down.

Drinking a glass of water before a meal will also prevent you from overeating – it makes you feel fuller.

Use Green Tea to Boost Your Metabolism

Green tea has been a stable of cultures for centuries due to its numerous medicinal purposes. But recently, attention has been focused on its ability to boost metabolism and, therefore, promote weight loss.

Green tea boosts metabolism by way of an antioxidant compound called catechins. Along with the natural caffeine, catechins regulate body fat and even help to prevent future weight gain by way of a complicated physiological process.

In this process, the sympathetic nervous system becomes stimulated. This causes the body to increases it's sensitivity to insulin. The combination of catechins and caffeine interferes with enzymes which target the body's regulation of energy as well as fat storage.

After a series of cellular chain reactions has occurred, the body's level of noradrenaline is massively increased which ultimately leads to fat being burned off at an accelerated rate. One of the main areas targeted for this fat elimination is visceral fat, or fat around the midsection.

It also lowers LDL, or "bad" cholesterol.

Now – we're not talking the bottled sugary green tea stuff. We're talking about the stuff in a little bag that you pour hot water over, let sit for five minutes, and then drink. THAT is green tea. Not something pre-mixed.

How Extra Protein Helps You Lose Weight

Recently, there's been a lot of attention focused on increasing protein consumption, such as utilizing high-protein diets, to help you lose weight. But is it safe? Yes, if done correctly.

Increasing protein helps weight loss in a lot of ways. It helps you feel fuller, faster so you tend to eat less. Since protein is so satiating it helps you to maintain that full feeling longer. Venus members receive a suggested protein guideline each week when they use the Venus Factor Virtual Nutritionist program in conjunction with their current age, weight, and body measurements. Protein also helps build muscle, which burns more fat. The key here is to only consume the leanest forms of protein such as extra lean meats and salmon.

Extra protein also allows you to curb certain cravings which can be detrimental, such as sweets and carbs.

Increasing your protein intake helps promote weight loss due to the process of thermogenesis. This is the process by which calories are consumed because of the way the body processes nutrients. Thermogenesis occurs at higher levels from protein than from other types of nutrients.

But there is such a thing as having too much protein, which can cause liver and kidney problems. Talk to your doctor or a certified dietitian to determine your ideal intake.

THIRTEEN

Cooking in Bulk and Planning Ahead

One of the surest ways to eat unhealthy is being caught at mealtime with nothing to prepare. Losing weight then takes a back seat to the convenience of drive-thru. That's why cooking is bulk is the best answer to this problem.

When you cook in bulk, you eliminate several problems:

1. Not wanting to cook. Sometimes, you're just too tired to cook.
2. No time. With our busy schedules, we often get home too late to prepare a meal
3. Nothing to cook. Getting caught with no healthy food in the house isn't good
4. Being tempted to eat out. This never leads to healthy choices.
5. Having to cook when you don't feel well.

Anyone can cook in bulk if they plan accordingly. Instead of making a single serving, double or triple the ingredients. But make sure to divide and store the leftovers before you sit down.

This isn't an invitation to overeat!

There's no limit to what you can cook in bulk. When you're ready to eat, simply heat it up and enjoy.

Super make-ahead ideas for anyone (especially Venus members):

- Thaw and marinate bulk bags of chicken breasts with low fat Italian or Balsamic Vinaigrette dressing. Grill outside until done, then cool and store in the refrigerator for lunches and dinners all week long.

- Make large saucepans of starchy foods like rice and quinoa, use chicken broth instead of water for a better flavor. Seal tightly and use ½ cup and 1 cup servings for lunches and dinners all week.

- Chop an assortment of fresh non-starchy vegetables. Heat oven to 450 degrees. Cover a large baking sheet with non-stick foil. Spray with non-stick spray (I know you're using non-stick foil, stay with me here). Scatter vegetables on pan, and drizzle with 2 tablespoons EVOO (extra virgin olive oil). Also drizzle some balsamic salad dressing, 2 – 3 tablespoons. Place vegetables in oven for 20 minutes. Take them out, turn and stir with a spatula, and put back in the oven for 15 – 20 minutes. Remove from heat, and let cool. Store tightly sealed in the fridge, enjoy with lunches and dinners all week (yummy!). Suggested veggies – yellow squash, zucchini, mushrooms, carrots, grape tomatoes (cut in half), bell peppers if you like them.

FOURTEEN

Emotional eating

Emotional eating is one of the biggest saboteurs of losing weight. We emotionally eat when we're depressed, anxious, nervous or upset. Learning how to avoid it will allow you to be successful.

In order to overcome emotional eating you have to identify everything that triggers it. Keep a journal to record these times and reflect on them.

How to avoid emotional eating:

- Reduce stress in your life.
- Get plenty of sleep.
- Listen to music you enjoy.
- Surround yourself with friends: limit alone time when you can become depressed.
- Make time for yourself.
- Don't eat in front of the TV.
- Never eat something out of its original container.
- Make sure to have healthy snacks with you when you're away from home.
- Go walking when you're stressed or upset.

- Set realistic weight loss goals.

- Have a friend on standby who can motivate and encourage you.

- Dangle a reward in front of yourself to motivate you.

- When you feel the urge to eat, make yourself exercise for 15 minutes. This sidetracks your self-destructive thoughts.

- Only stock healthy foods. You can't eat it if it isn't there.

FIFTEEN

Tips and Tricks to be **NORMAL** When Eating Out

Even when we are trying to lose weight, we still enjoy eating out occasionally. But it's easy to have your efforts sabotaged by the enormous portions that are served in restaurants. However, you can still enjoy dining out if you simply split the meal first (with yourself, or with someone else).

As soon as the food comes to the table ask the served to bring you a to-go container. Your standard entrée in today's restaurants are so much larger than they were just a few short decades ago. While you should enjoy your food, you still don't want to undo everything that you've worked so hard to accomplish.

When the server brings you a container, divide the food up before you even take your first bite. This keeps you from being tempted to overeat. And don't rely on yourself to stop eating half way through the meal or before you know it, you'll be staring down at an empty plate. Divide the food up first and you will be able to enjoy the second half of the entrée at another meal.

If you AND your significant other are food conscious – split your meals as a rule! This is something that I've always done with my sweetie, and it makes for a more romantic evening when we can sit next to each other and eat off of the same plate.

Other Quick Tips:

- When you order a sandwich – lose half of the bread right away. Just take it off! Peel off the good stuff, and tuck it under or on top of the remainder of the sandwich.

- Order the sandwich without bread – many places will do this, especially with folks following the so-called "gluten-free" fad. (Don't get me started – my daughter has Celiac disease, she really doesn't CHOOSE to be gluten-free, it chose her!)

- When asked "what side do you want with that?" – ask for steamed vegetables. Or no side at all. Or a side salad with balsamic vinaigrette (on the side, so that you can control how much oil goes on your salad).

- Get out your calorie counting app on your smart phone – and find foods based on the restaurant's name! I've been asked to go out to eat on the fly quite a few times, and this is my "go to" to decide what I'm going to eat! I look for meals or dishes that are below what I decide is my calorie limit for that meal – and have that. Simple.

- Order a side salad – and ask if you can have some grilled shrimp or grilled chicken on that. They will typically give you three to four ounces of protein, sometimes up to five ounces. You might also have a piece of bread, if it's not dipped and rolled and saturated in butter (I know, I want it too, but maybe on a splurge day!)

Last note on eating out – if you're meeting friends for a drink – have a drink! But count the calories. Know what you're having – here's a list of lifestyle friendly choices:

- Red Wine – 5 ounces – 100 calories / 2 grams carbs
- White Wine – 5 ounces – 100 calories / 2 grams carbs
- Scotch – 1.5 ounces – 104 calories / 0 grams carbs
- Vodka – 1.5 ounces – 104 calories / 0 grams carbs
- Light Beer – 12 ounces – 108 calories / 6 grams carbs (some light beers are lower in calories than others)
- Draft Beer – 12 ounces – 144 calories / 13.2 grams carbs
- Manhattan – 3.3 ounces – 153 calories / 3.6 grams carbs
- Martini – 2.2 ounces – 135 calories / 3.6 grams carbs

SIXTEEN

It's Okay To Feel Hungry

It's really – really okay to feel hungry. Seriously. That little twinge, that little growl – that's normal. It's not going to "kill" you. If you're reading this book – you're not walking around because you don't have food – you've had too much.

One of my favorite novels that I read as a young woman - revolved around a female character that was born fat, raised fat, and had accepted herself as fat. To break away from her boring fat life, she took a year to live in Paris with a widow and her two daughters. Her room and board was paid for by her family – but "board", which means meals, was very different than what she'd been raised on. Her meals were tiny, miniscule, a fraction of what she was used to eating. She cried in her room, because she was starving, she was hungry. And she didn't have any spending money to go buy the pastries and sweets that she'd consoled herself with when at home.

But after months of this reduced eating lifestyle… the unhappy young woman – emerged a much smaller, slimmer version of herself. Yep – she wasn't fat because she was "born" to be fat – she'd just eaten too much. And her one mantra moving on – "stay just a little hungry".

43

I loved that story. But the truth is — we can all stand to be a little hungry, sometimes. It's okay.

Now, "out of control — about to eat your neighbor's sunburned arm like a zombie and you have a headache" hungry — yeah, that's not cool. Eat a piece of string cheese. Now.

SEVENTEEN

Building Muscle Can Help You Burn Fat 24/7

Pound for pound, muscle weights the same as fat. But each requires a different amount of energy.

Research shows us that the more muscle your body has the higher your metabolism will be. This results in an increases burn rate of stored fat. Does this mean that you need to be a bodybuilder in order to burn fat? No. But it does mean that an individual who as more muscle will have a higher metabolism compared to a lean individual with a lower muscle mass.

But the fat burning doesn't end there. Even after a workout, muscle continues to burn even more fat. Muscle requires a greater amount of energy, energy derived from stored supplies. As muscle repairs itself during rest, the "burn" is still occurring.

Even at rest, our bodies need energy to maintain their numerous systems and to perform their multiple functions. Muscle accelerates that burning and reduces the amount of fat being stored.

And it makes your clothes fit better. You KNOW it does!

EIGHTEEN

The Role of Good Sleep in Weight Loss

Getting a good night's sleep does more than make you refreshed. It also helps with weight loss. When your body does not enough sleep, several key chemical reactions take place that affect your weight:

First, the body release the stress hormone, cortisol, in response. Cortisol can cause you to eat more out of anxiety.

Second, the body's levels of the hormones ghrelin are increased, and leptin levels are decreased. Both hormones are responsible for maintaining feelings of fullness after a meal and for helping to control hunger pains. Produced in the gastrointestinal tract, ghrelin is what stimulates appetite. When sleep is deprived, it causes ghrelin levels to increase and you feel hungrier.

When we lose sleep, our level of leptin, which is manufactured in our fat cells, goes down. Optimal levels of leptin signal the brain that we're full. When this level is down, the brain isn't notified and we tend to overeat.

Alone, each one of these actions can lead to weight gain. But together, the consequences to our weight are multiplied exponentially.

So, what does this mean? Don't stay up all night. Get enough sleep. How much is enough? Enough that you don't keep hitting the snooze button for an hour every morning. Aim for seven hours, eight if you can.

NINETEEN

Eating On Smaller Dishes

We all know the key to losing weight is taking in less calories than we need. A good way to do that is by fooling the brain using smaller plates.

Food is visual. Some overeat because the food is readily available to them in abundance. Others overeat so as not to waste food. Smaller plates eliminate both problems because you are limiting the amount of food in front of you.

We all love to fill our plate at mealtime. Many choose not to diet because they don't want to be deprived. A smaller plate allows the mind to think that we aren't depriving it of food. But the real trick involves timing. Once your plate is clean, sit back and give yourself 15 minutes before returning for seconds. It takes the brain that long to register food once it is consumed.

It defeats the purpose of a smaller plate if food is piled too high. Keep it no more than an inch high all across the plate.

TWENTY

Eating Too Quickly

Eating too quickly causes weight gain for one simple reason: you tend to overeat.

When you eat too fast you aren't giving your stomach enough time to notify your brain that it is full. How long does it take food to register in the brain? From 15 to 20 minutes. If you're eating too quickly, you can consume a considerable amount of calories in that amount of time before your brain can tell you to put down your fork.

For some, eating quickly is psychological. They know their body only has about 20 minutes from the first bite to signal that the stomach is full. Eating faster allows them to enjoy more of their favorite foods in the same amount of time than if they ate at a normal pace.

How do you stop eating fast? Put down your fork between each bite. Chew each bite slowly and at least twenty times before swallowing. Sip water between bites. Start your meals with lean proteins, vegetables and fruits. Save the carbs and fat for later - if there's time.

TWENTY ONE

If You Hit A Weight Loss Plateau, Do Something Different With Your Exercise Routine

Anyone who has ever tried it will tell you that it's very difficult to stay motivated when you're trying to lose weight. What makes matters worse is when you hit a plateau.

Plateaus are notorious for popping up just as we are beginning to see results from our efforts. Not only are they incredibly frustrating, but if you don't rectify the solution soon you'll lose interest and faith in working out just as quickly.

Over time, your body begins to adapt to your exercise routine. It adjusts to the demands that you are placing on it. Eventually, you will hit a point where your efforts don't seem to be paying off. When that happens, you have to confuse the body by changing your routine.

Keep a record of your exercise routine, so you know exactly what to change, and by how much. Increase the amount of time you exercise. If you typically walk on a treadmill, try aerobics instead. Add something new, and take something away. Do something to drastically alter your workout, and shake your body back to losing weight. If another plateau hits, change it again.

TWENTY TWO

Cardio vs. Strength Training

So – you're doing this thing, you're going to eat less, and you're going to lose weight, and then maintain your weight loss when you get where you want to be. But, hey, maybe you want to eat a little MORE than totally less – so you're going to exercise, right? Right!

So, what kind of exercise should you do? Should you invest in Jane Fonda sweats and become a cardio bunny? Or just dig out your old running shoes and take a morning run every day? Or is weight-lifting going to be a better option? Because there's all kinds of exercising to do. Too many choices – maybe just sleep in? (Kidding – keep reading).

If you are in an epic battle with your scale, cardio is your best choice - cardio burns more calories than strength training.

However, cardio doesn't do much for your muscles. In one Penn State study, dieters lost 21 pounds whether they performed cardio or strength training. But for the cardio group, six of those pounds came from muscle, while the strength trainers lost almost pure fat—and probably fit into their skinny jeans better because of it.

Why do you think that is? Strength training is the best way to build more muscle. And for every pounds of muscle you gain, you can expect to burn an extra 50 calories a day without moving a single one of those muscles. (Hey – didn't we say something at the beginning of this chapter about wanting to eat more? Now – granted, the 50 calories just MAY be an overstatement by the LYING, CHEATING DIET INDUSTRY... but still, biology and mathematics reasonably say you DO need more energy when you have more muscle mass. Just don't assume you can have an ice cream sundae every day!)

That doesn't mean that you should retire your running shoes or your biking jersey, though—especially if you're a stress eater. Cardio is one of the best ways to conquer stress, which is a waistline-wrecker all by itself (you may remember that nasty hormone cortisol, the one that is linked to high stress levels that makes us want to eat more). The best solution? A combination of both strength training AND cardio.

If you can do some cardio on three days a week, and then do strength training for two to three days a week – that's probably the most perfect combination you can do. Time crunched? Go for the strength training with a five minute cardio warmup.

How much cardio? Whatever feels good to you. You really don't start sweating until about 20 minutes into that workout (common sense), so start there. Or end there. And it also depends on your time constraints, and your lifestyle. If your job has you on your feet eight hours a day walking around, I'd say you've got your cardio in.

You might want to do 20 minutes of sustained activity at some point, but you're already pretty active – and might ALREADY need an extra 100 – 200 calories a day.

How much weight lifting? Over the course of two workouts, you want to hit all of your major muscle groups with two to three sets of repetitions. You'll notice above that I mentioned THREE weight lifting sessions per week. So you'll be constantly straddling muscle groups across weeks – and this is a good thing. It allows you to tear down the muscle tissue, and it allows adequate time for the tissue to heal and grow.

Will you get big and bulky and look like a guy? Only if you are a guy. Sorry, ladies – it takes a lot of guy hormones to bulk up. You're not going to look like a huge female body builder. You're going to look very sleek and toned. You'll look nice!

How do you find out what kind of strength training exercises to do? You need to find a good personal trainer, or a weight-lifting program to walk you through that. Venus Factor has great three day a week weight-lifting plans with video demonstrations – it's great, and it's included in the onetime price mentioned at the beginning of the book. Don't forget to UNSUBSCRIBE from the endless e-mails you'll get afterwards!

Okay – now for the problem children – you know who you are. I'll try to address some special situations here:

1) **Road Warriors** – these folks travel a lot for work. They typically excuse themselves from exercise because it's just too inconvenient. Baloney. If it's important, you'll do it. Hotels have gyms, go use them. Lace up your running shoes, and run around the parking lot fifty time (yes, I really have done that before). Pack resistance bands in your suitcase, and do your strength training by stepping on the band and pushing and pulling against the resistance. You can also purchase an anchor that loops around the hinge of your hall doorframe, and anchor the resistance band to that, and push and pull against that.

2) **New moms** – been there, too. First thing – WAIT FOR YOUR DOCTOR TO SAY ITS OKAY TO EXERCISE. Seriously. Your body just went through major trauma – let it heal, girl! Once you've got the okay – take it easy. You still have a lot of hormones running through you that loosened up your ligaments so that you could do one huge amazing thing – until those hormones go away, you run a higher risk of injuring your joints and muscles. Go slow on your cardio, go light on your weight lifting. And rest. Now – you're no longer a "new mom" at around four months post-partum – get back in the groove, and hit it hard! I know that you're tired, the baby sometimes keeps you up all night, and then you have to work the next day. But you need to take care of YOU. Ask for help, ask someone to watch that baby while you take a walk, do a DVD workout, escape to the gym for an hour. If you can't find

someone to help you, find a gym with a nursery that you TRUST. For your own sanity, GET SOME EXERCISE!!!

3) **Special needs** – what if you're wheelchair bound? You've got some issues that are beyond my scope. But if you do have use of your arms – you can exercise. I know – because I've watched handcycle athletes participate in half ironman triathlons for the last twelve years. They exercise – so can you. Other folks with debilitating painful conditions – I got it. You're in pain. But if you can walk – you can walk – go do that. You don't have to speed walk. And you can probably lift something, even a one pound weight or a water bottle will do. Lift that.

4) **Time challenged people** – you don't have time to exercise. I know – I've been there too. And if you really want to do it, you will. You will DELEGATE some of your responsibilities to someone else, and take care of YOURSELF. If you do not take care of YOURSELF, you will BURN OUT and GO CRAZY. And really, nobody likes crazy you. They like cool, calm, happy you. Go exercise, and be the best YOU possible!

TWENTY THREE

On Eating Fiber – and Why You Want To

Fiber – yes, we're talking the stuff that old folks stir into their orange juice so that they can be "regular". Hopefully, you're getting enough by choosing to eat some vegetables and fruits in your calorie budget.

But – sometimes, those high fiber foods end up falling off of our "foods of choice" when we're counting calories, especially fruits. Why? Because they're higher in carbohydrates, and higher in sugar content. Even so, for their size and weight, they're a good choice because the bulk of their weight is water, and fiber.

What happens when we don't get enough fiber in our diets? I think most of us know – but I'll spell it out. We don't get adequate and satisfying bowel movements. Our gut may feel uncomfortably full at times, and we may feel bloated. Visiting the bathroom may be uncomfortable, and feel like a waste of time – because nothing is happening.

So, what's the solution? Obviously, eat more fiber. But…what if we don't want to "spend" calories on those food? Try a supplement. The bad news is that the supplements don't really give you that much fiber. Sorry! But you can use a drinking water additive that's clear and tasteless, and comes in handy packets that are portable. Those have about 3 grams of fiber (you want around 25 grams of fiber per day to be – regular). Using a tracker like MyFitnessPal will total up your fiber and give you a clue if you're NOT getting close to where you should be.

Other things to do – if you're eating breads, rice and pastas, check the labels for the ones with higher fiber content. Every gram counts!

In Conclusion

So, we're at the end of the book. What have you learned? Hopefully, you've learned that YOU already knew the answer to how to lose the weight and keep it off. You've just been brainwashed by the diet and fitness industry into thinking that YOU weren't doing it right.

They've been feeding you lies, and telling you that you can eat more food, but in reality, you can't. And you secretly knew this, but have been in denial.

You've also read through some valuable tips that you may have already read somewhere else. Do these things.

What are your first steps to get started, if you haven't gotten started? Okay, I'll spell it out for you. I do love a good checklist!

1) Determine your BMR (Basal Metabolic Rate) How? Open an internet browser, and go to the MyFitnessPal BMR Calculator. Input your CURRENT information – it will tell you how many calories you need to maintain your CURRENT weight with NO exercise.

2) How active are you? Sedentary means you have an office job and don't exercise. You're not really active at all – you don't need any extra calories to function (being stressed doesn't count). Say your job has you on your feet a lot – you may need an extra 100 calories a day to MAINTAIN. Maybe a little more. Say that you coach your kid's soccer team three days a week, and run for 30 minutes three days a week. You might need an extra 300 calories a day to MAINTAIN.

3) <u>Add the calories from #1 and #2 together</u>. THAT total is your MAINTENANCE CALORIE BUDGET. In order to MAINTAIN your current weight – you should average around THAT over several days. (Do you want me to apologize? It's not my fault – we've ALL been brainwashed, it sucks that we've been told we can eat more, unfortunately, we can't).

4) <u>Eat less than your body needs</u> - Now, in order to LOSE weight, we need to go seriously BELOW that number. SERIOUSLY BELOW that number, at least six days a week most weeks. Let's look at a real person as an example (she's not real, I'm making her up):

Sally is 38, is five feet three inches tall, weighs 165. She has three kids in two different schools, works in accounting at the plant across town, and her kids are in Tae Kwon Do and soccer year round.

Sally plugs in her numbers, and finds out her BMR is 1398. Wow, she says, and the last diet she was on had her eating 1500 calories a day! Until she couldn't stand it anymore and gave up again, as she went through the drive through at KFC yet again.

But wait – Sally makes it a habit to walk around the soccer field and listen to Pitbull while the kids are playing and practicing. And at the Tae Kwon Do studio, there's an old exercise bike that she'll hop on because she's bored and the parent chairs are uncomfortable. Plus, at the plant that she works at, she has a walking group and they walk on their breaks and get about three quarters of a mile in when the weather is good. All total, Sally probably burns an extra 300 calories a day with her active lifestyle, which brings up her approximate total to around 1700 calories a day to MAINTAIN HER CURRENT WEIGHT.

So – losing weight. How low can we go? That's up to you – but you want to undercut your MAINTENANCE CALORIE BUDGET by at least 500 calories. Yes, I said it. 500 – or more. HARD LIMIT – don't go below 1000 calories a day. Seriously –

that's what the medical industry calls a VLC Diet – Very Low Calorie. At that low a calorie intake level, you need to be monitored by a doctor. Don't go that low.

1000 calories a day? Seriously? Yes, seriously. Now, if you're a VERY active person, or have a VERY LARGE muscle mass, you may need to adjust that higher. If you're a very large person with a lot of fat reserves – you do not. 1000 calories a day will be a huge shock to your system for a few days. But you'll get used to it.

EVERY DAY? Just 1000 calories? Most days, yes. But one day a week, eat your Maintenance Calories, or a little above. KEEP COUNTING THOSE CALORIES. That extra 500 or 800 calories isn't going to make you gain weight. It may slow your loss for a couple of days, but you won't gain.

How much will you lose by following a program like this?

How much do you need to lose? By restricting calories, you will lose weight. As long as you keep doing it. Period.

How much weight should you lose?

Seriously? You're asking me? Ask your doctor, go find some insurance table. When you get there, you'll know.

Can I eat more food when I reach my ideal or desired weight?

You can eat your MAINTENANCE CALORIE BUDGET when you want to MAINTAIN your CURRENT weight (Oh, and guess what, you need to go RE-DO your BMR. That's right, you'll weigh less). When you want to LOSE weight – go back down to 1000 calories, until you are back at your goal.

Can I go through the drive-thru at KFC and eat food from there?

Well, ask yourself - does the food at KFC have calories? Can you find those calories in your MyFitnessPal app? Do you have enough calories in your Calorie Budget today? Then yes, you can eat at

KFC. Let's examine. Crispy Chicken Strips are 380 calories. Corn cob is around 100, depending on how big it is. 480 calories – that's around half of my calories for the day. As long as my other meal is reasonable, and I have just one snack today – yes, KFC is a decent choice.

When I find myself in a bind – colleagues from work ask me to lunch at the last minute, I hit up MyFitnessPal with the restaurant name, and I scroll through looking for calorie values, until I find something that fits my budget. And I decide right then – I'll have that. I may stash the brown bag lunch I already have prepared and eat it tomorrow – but yes, go out with your friends, and eat at restaurants. It's really okay. Just choose wisely.

I've said all I have to say – if you have more questions about Back 2 Basics, e-mail me:

wanda@mommywisesup.com

If your questions do not involve common sense – I may knock some sense into you. Just sayin'.

About the Author

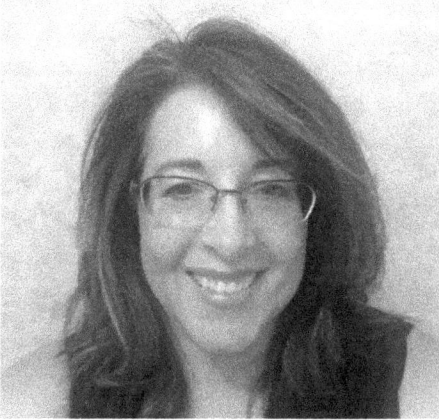

Wanda Bailey has engaged in public speaking gigs for thirty years, and creating training programs for that long, as well! She's had many blessings in her life - she's worked in accounting and payroll, she's been a music director at two different churches. She's worked in staffing, web design and marketing, and was also a nanny! In her early twenties, she worked for Weight Watchers International as a Leader.

She's traveled all over the United States of America doing software training, both in person, remotely, and in video presentations. She studied in Mexico as a teenager, and has visited Canada, Ireland, Germany and Austria.

She has four children - the youngest is almost finished with high school.

Visit her website – www.mommywisesup.com for information on what else she does!

Other books by Wanda at time of publication

Divorce Blueprint – Your Advice Handbook From Start to Recovery

Going Gluten Free – From Gluten Sensitivity to Celiac Disease – Changing Your Eating Lifestyle

Do You Want To Write A Book?

Everyone has a book in them – are you ready to publish it? Please visit www.dragongempublishing.com for some help. We offer self-publishing information, and done-for-you publishing packages.